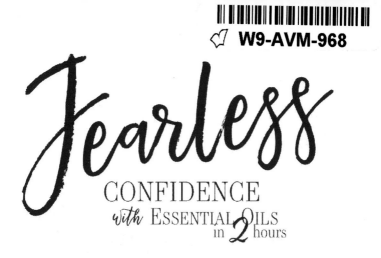

Fearless

CONFIDENCE
with ESSENTIAL OILS
in **2** hours

Sarah Harnisch
YOUNG LIVING DIAMOND

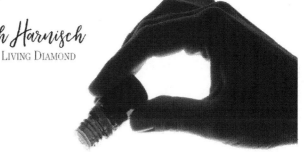

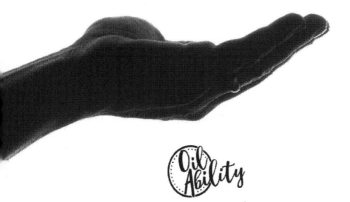

Oil Ability

Layout and cover design: Jeremy Holden (JeremyHolden.me)

Cover photo: Josh Puccio (www.joshuapuccio.com)

Editing team: Maria Waddell and Trina Holden

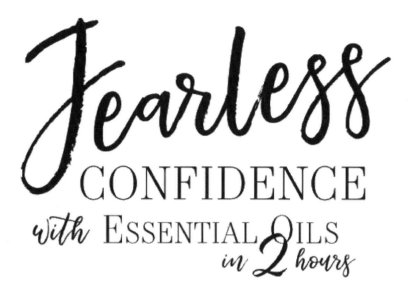

Fearless CONFIDENCE with ESSENTIAL OILS in 2 hours

Hey! Welcome to essential oils! If you just got your Young Living Starter kit in the mail and it's a little intimidating, or you have had your kit for a while, but it's collecting dust because you don't know what to do with it--this book is for you!

Maybe you're eyeing a kit, but you're not sure you would use it. You love the smell of Peppermint, but have no idea how to incorporate it into a daily routine. This little book is for you, too.

You're probably thinking (as I did!) --"There are so many books about essential oils! Where do I start? How to I get to know my oils and how to use them properly?" If you're worried about wasting your investment, or making a mistake, or if these little drops will stack up to what you've been using for years...

If you love the idea of becoming an oiler, but are overwhelmed...

It's ok.

You're in the right place. In the next two hours, I will carry you far from those places. *I was you*. I have walked this path. I came from the darkest past, filled with so many toxic chemicals that it caused monthly brain bleeds. And I learned slowly how to move from that place.

Now, my life is completely different. I have had all your questions and all your thoughts and all your doubts. Today is the day we eradicate fear together. Together we are going to cross the gap between not feeling confident about using essential oils to a life filled sunup to sundown with essential oils. It's a toxic chemical free lifestyle. All it takes is a little training and encouragement, and that's why I'm here.

My name is Sarah Harnisch. I am a Young Living Diamond and an essential oils addict, and I'm going to help you grow confident with oils and

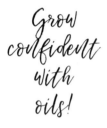

get the most out of your starter kit. I have been using and sharing oils for three years, and I have seen people fall in love and become die-hard oilers. But I've also seen starter kits re-sold online, still wrapped in plastic. It all boils down to one reason: they never knew the treasure inside the box.

Why all this excitement about 11 oils? Because it has the power to alter your life. It is a course correction. It is a complete perspective shift on how you take care of yourself and your family. By taking tiny, baby steps into a natural lifestyle (at a pace you choose), you can dramatically change your exposure to poisons and toxic chemicals.

Oils aren't just weird bottles that only certified aromatherapists know how to use. They have been around since the dawn of time (and used by millions of people without certifications). If they are a fad, they are a fad with a track record that spans millennia. They are also your gateway to change how you care for your family.

The reality is that most of us fall somewhere between the crunchy enthusiast that sleeps on bamboo sheets and eats leaves and nothing else; and the fast-food dining connoisseur who lives in a chemical cesspool. Most of us want to do better for our families—but we aren't sure what that looks like, or if we actually have time. And it seems like the information out there would take a lifetime to learn.

When we get oils in our hands, we love the *idea* of them, but aren't sure what to *do* with them. I was in that category three years ago. I had zero exposure to pure essential oils. But I got my kit and I began to experiment, playing with the oils. I built a massive team and a massive income with just one thing: passion. And now I've put together a guide to teach you how to play with your kit. It's called *Fearless* because we're about to annihilate your fear of oils.

I'm going to walk you through, step by step, how to get to know your oils until you can't imagine life without them. I'll train you how to make oils your focal point, not your afterthought. If you accept my 10 Challenges and truly walk through them over and over and over again until they become normal for you, be prepared to eliminate worry about how you care for your spouse and kids. You will walk with confidence through your home, knowing you have made a simple swap of toxic chemicals at every turn that will impact your family in a positive way.

This book isn't about pretty bottles that smell good. It's about changing the way you look at every product you buy. It's to train your eyes to hunt for dangers in your home and teaching you to label read, so you can spot poison in your cabinets and start making the best choices for your family.

WHY START WITH OILS?

Because everything else has a larger learning curve. Oils are the bridge to natural health. Young Living oils come ready to go, right out of the bottle. There is no science you need to master. There are no fancy techniques to learn. The work has been done for you by God creating incredible plants. Every day, all over the world, the experts on Young Living's farms are capturing the power of the plants and putting them into a bottle with their amazing seed to seal guarantee. Distilling oils is not a skill you need to master. You just need to learn to play with the kit.

Other natural living techniques take more time and effort. If you're learning fermenting, you must find cultures and be comfortable having weird things growing on your counter. If you're learning homeopathy, you must learn to source, harvest, dry, boil, and bottle herbs and tinctures. If you're learning organic gardening, you must learn pH and soil and composting and where and how to plant. With oils, you open the bottle and run with it. It requires no degree. Oils are simple and they work.

Perhaps up until this point you haven't had a lot of interest in what's in your cabinets or in your diet. You figure if you're not eating fast food several times a week and you're not a soda or junk food addict, you're in decent shape. In this little book, I will challenge you and encourage you to kick it up a notch and make the shift in every single product you use, eat, or wear. You are the gatekeeper of your house. It's up to you to protect what's in those four walls. No one is looking out for your family but you. It's time to take this far beyond a starter kit, and into every room of your home. Are you ready for a game-changer? Are you ready to take the next step? Are you ready to take this seriously? You have already made the investment in a Premium Starter kit. Now it's time to show you where this goes. I promise you, it's good.

I will shoot straight with you: there is a learning curve to oiling, but it's not because it's hard. It's because you must untrain yourself from reaching for other options. You have to untrain all your habits, and untrain all your connections to old smells and things you've used for years. You have to be willing to lose social esteem—not everyone will think you're sane. But it's not as hard if you know your "why".

My "why" is that I am tired of what the industry tells me is safe. I am tired of government approvals of products that should never, ever be in anyone's home. I'm tired of wiping my counters down with bottles that say they're poisonous and cannot be consumed. I'm weary of smelling like toxic chemicals when I wash my hair, and eating foods that make me groggy because they are processed with synthetic vitamins and chemically-processed, fake ingredients that don't resemble anything my grandparents would have seen on their tables. I am tired of walking through the grocery store and getting a headache when I pass the cleaning supplies aisle. I'm tired of a toxic lifestyle, and I'm saying no to dangerous chemicals in my home. My family will no longer be exposed to anything I can't control.

I am pretty sure you're on the same path with me, because you wouldn't have your starter kit sitting on a shelf! So let's learn together, side by side, step by step, piece by piece, at your pace. That's why this book is tiny and digestible. It's your getting-started place.

This little book is probably a bit different from what you've seen before, because it's not an encyclopedia of plant names and origins hundreds of pages long, and it's not a simple flyer with lists of uses for the starter kit. (Those are both great tools that I use in my home! But this book serves a different purpose). For the first time, I am explaining what it looks like to be someone who uses essential oils daily. In one sitting you will go from a non-oiler or passive oiler to one that's passionate and trying new things each day with purpose. If you can get past the habits of reaching for the familiar, old things you're used to, you're on the road to cleaning out the cabinets of your home. Every oil you use is a toxic chemical you're not using. Whether you take this book and explode and detox your entire house, or whether you just apply a few principles; we have grown together, and you have done an excellent job.

What makes me qualified to tell you how to use your kit? I have studied at multiple aromatherapy schools and hold six certifications in aromatherapy—from Biblical Aromatherapy to Aroma Chemistry. I have instructed thousands in mass classes across the country. But my best qualification is pain. It's my past. It's where I came from. It's the result of my poor decisions. If showing you my mistakes inspires you to make some changes, then this book was worth it for me. Walk with me for a few minutes while I share the very beginning of the story of how I found essential oils.

HOW MAKING A SWAP SAVED MY LIFE

I used to be a migraine sufferer. I have gotten my life back because of simple swaps I made in my food and in my cabinets. Swapping out toxins is not a game. You cannot do what you were called and created to do if you have lost your health. Your talents and gifts and drive and creativity and purpose mean nothing if you are suffering. The problem is that most people don't make the connection between the way that they feel and the toxic products in their home.

I had my first migraine headache when I was 12 years old. I bore them for 24 solid years— through the birth of all five of my kids, and through 20 years of anchoring radio network news at 4 a.m. I bore them through seven hours of homeschooling my kids every day for 15 years.

My migraines would last ten days on a bell curve, every single month, following the ebb and flow of my hormone cycle. They would start with photosensitivity and numbness on one side of my face, and would progress to debilitating, severe pain down the right side of my head and face. My body responded with tremoring and diarrhea. My face would droop on one side and I would drop things I tried to carry with my right hand. By day four or five, I was curled into a ball on my bed for most of the day, gripping my knees in agonizing pain. I'd wake up, anchor news, come home at 10:00 or 11:00 a.m. and stay in a dark room all day long, writhing in pain. I was a non-existent mom for three or four days a month during the worst of it. Many months, I would have my husband drive me to the emergency room for what they called the migraine cocktail: a pain medication, an anti-nausea medication, and an anti-inflammatory drug given intravenously to stop the cycle of vomiting from the pain so I would not get dehydrated.

By the time I was 30, I had seen 13 different neurologists and been on 16 families of migraine medicines. Each one had a different side effect. Some made my throat swell to the point that I had to make a visit to the emergency room. Others made my headaches worse. One time, I started a new med right before our family went to see an action movie. Three minutes into it, I was throwing my hands up in front of my face, thinking the actors were kicking me. We had to leave—I was hallucinating. Some medicines made me gain 30 or 40 pounds (I normally weigh 125!) And the last group of drugs were narcotics that turned me into a vegetable, where I slept all day long, numbed from the pain. None of those were good options for me.

Once I started doing yearly MRI's, we found something terrible. Every month I would have a migraine, the vessels on my brain would swell, and cause tiny pin-prick bleeds on my brain. Each year I'd get a new scan, and we would compare them from year to year, and every year I had 30-40 new dark black spots on the surface of my brain from the bleeding. I was losing my memory. It was causing traumatic damage. And I was at risk for a catastrophic stroke—at age 30.

What was my diet like? I didn't think it had anything to do with my problem. I just wanted a pill to make it better. I ate like an average American—fast food a few days a week, processed food in my cabinets. I made my kids foods out of a box loaded with dyes and I warmed up frozen processed meals. I fed them enriched bread every day with fake vitamins. I drank soda pop by the half gallon each day. I sprayed my counters and windows and bathrooms with chemical cleaner. I mopped my floor with chemicals. I brushed my teeth with chemicals and washed my hair with chemicals and washed my clothes with chemicals. I figured it was all safe. It was all on a shelf at the store.

When I was 30, the migraines had gotten so bad that I was sent to a special headache clinic in Rochester, New York. They did the most comprehensive study I'd ever had. The doctor wanted me on six medications a day: one for pain, one for swelling, one to break the cycle of vomiting, a steroid, and two other medications to counteract the side effects of the first four.

I got home and lined all the bottles up on my counter and did something I didn't usually do: I started researching. Up until that point, I'd taken everything for face value. If it was in a store, it was safe. If it was on TV, it was safe. For the first time in my life, I started to question everything. Taking pills every two hours for the rest of my life to prevent a stroke—when I was only 30 years old—was daunting. My kids were 0, 2, 4, 6, and 8. I wanted to be around for them. I wanted to make sure this was the road I should be taking.

The first medication I looked up scared me. It was the steroid. There were over four pages of warnings that came with it. Most were heart-related. I was born with a level 5 heart murmur and a tricuspid regurgitation (a large valve in my heart that backflows). It seemed that if I took this medication, I could put myself in a risk category for a heart attack, especially if I was on it long-term. I took the bottles back to my neurologist and asked him what to do. He said, "if it was me, I'd take the medicine. If I had to choose between a stroke or a heart attack, I'd choose the heart attack. If you have a heart attack, you're dead immediately. If you have a stroke, you will be able to watch your kids grow up, but never be able to communicate with them. To me, that would be worse."

> "If it was in a store, I thought it was safe."

I remember walking out of his office thinking, "Who are you to decide that for me??" None of the options looked good. After I met with the neurologist, I contacted a good friend of mine, Trina Holden, who had written a great book called *Real Fast Food,* about swapping out the food that you eat (you can find it at trinaholden.com). I asked her what to do. She told me my diet was terrible—and diet was everything. I rolled my eyes. (I am a news anchor by trade—and naturally critical!) I could not imagine that changing the way that I ate would eradicate brain bleeds. Everyone else ate the way that I ate without visible consequences. I couldn't live on salads my whole life. I had every excuse in the book. But also, I'D

ALREADY TRIED IT. I had tried to eat well, sometimes for a month, and saw no change. I cut soda for six months at a time, and the migraines were still there. I had cut Chinese food, MSG, coffee, and preservatives and they were still there. It didn't work.

But as I thought it through for weeks... what did I have to lose? I'd already tried nearly every drug created for migraines. I'd been to neurologists in multiple states. I had been to a headache clinic. I had gone through years of MRI's. I was at a dead end—a fork in the road. Either I went with the way I'd been trained all my life and trusted the system, or I stepped out of what I knew and tried something radically different: a total lifestyle change. I decided that if a lifestyle change got rid of the migraines, it was worth it. I didn't see how something so simple could be the key, but I was willing to try.

I want you to know that my husband, John, and I are not against the medical system. We take our kids for yearly well-child checks. There are thousands of lives saved every day by the men and women doing surgeries and taking care of people. This is simply the story of my own personal path, and the choice I had to make when it was narrowed down to a pile of drugs every two hours or a lifestyle change. I believe medicine serves a valuable purpose, and there are many amazing doctors and nurses on my oils team that I deeply trust. This is simply my personal story and conviction, and the road that ultimately led me to oils. I didn't have peace at the only path that seemed open to me. If you are on medication, I strongly encourage you to speak with your doctor before making any changes to what you're doing.

For the first time in my life, I chose a lifestyle change. I was raised on boxed and canned and frozen everything, so this was a big shift for me. I had to erase all I'd ever known about food and toxic chemicals.

I didn't see how something so simple could be the key, but I was willing to try.

I started with a book called *Gut and Psychology Syndrome (GAPS)*. GAPS isn't for everyone. I'm convinced it's the most masochistic diet out there, and by far the hardest thing I've ever done. I wanted gut healing. Trina told me if I heal the gut, I heal the head. The head was what I was going for, so I started with the gut. There was a six-step system for detoxing my body.

I started with bone broth, made from organic chickens (basically soup). I advanced to new foods each week and skin tested them on my arm to see if my system was ready to handle it. I had to cut all sugar, all gluten, and all dairy. I lived on GAPS for five full years.

The premise of GAPS is that the body was designed to heal itself. But every single day we are putting things into it that prevent it from healing. The body must stop the healing process and go deal with those things, storing them, purging them, or using what they can from them. If we remove the foods that make our body work so hard, add fermented foods to pull all the nutrients out of what we're eating so we heal faster, and get on a fantastic probiotic to repopulate the good bacteria army in our gut, we have set up the perfect storm for our body to recover stand on its own two feet. I didn't know it then, but that's exactly what oils do. They don't heal the body. They set up the perfect storm for the body to heal itself— coming alongside and supporting the body. It's really neat to see.

AFter just one month on GAPS, I had no pain. For the first time in 24 years, I went 30 solid days without the debilitating, writhing pain of a migraine. The second month I was on it, the numbness and drooping on my right side left my body was gone. I had never officially had a stroke during all those years of migraines, but I was at an elevated risk for one. I once asked the neurologist how I knew if it was a stroke or a migraine. He told me, "If the migraine goes away, and you still have lost function on the right side of your body, come in here as quickly as you can. You have had a stroke, and the sooner you get here the better." For more than a decade, I wondered every month if that was going to be the month that the I'd have a catastrophic stroke. I sat there looking at my kids, wondering if I would be able to see them grow up.

By month three on GAPS, every migraine symptom I had for 24 years was completely gone. My skin cleared up. Inflammation in my body was gone. I felt like a totally different person, simply by changing the way that I ate. It has been five years since my last migraine. For five straight years, despite the stress of moving across the country, raising an autistic son, and homeschooling all five of the kids; the migraines have never returned. It wasn't my stress level causing my health problems. It was the things I exposed myself to, willingly, day after day after day. My body had enough. It had rebelled.

One thing that GAPS did for me was that it made me a very good label reader. When you can't have any gluten or things that can mimic gluten—like arrowroot powder, tapioca flour, or potato flour—you get good at reading the labels on the products you're buying. I pushed it a step farther and started reading more labels. If I could not handle ice cream or sandwiches, which seem harmless, I wanted to know about the dangers of my bright blue dish soap. My family washes their dishes with it, then eats off those same plates that still smell like chemicals. I wanted to know about the hazards of laundry soap. My kid's clothes rub on their skin all day long after being washed in toxic soap, then they breathe the smell of the chemicals from their clothes all night long as they outgas in their closet. I can smell chemicals from the laundry soap on other people's clothes as I pass them, hours and sometimes days after the clothes have been washed. I wanted to know about my counter cleaner that says, "Poisonous, do not consume." I use it to sanitize my butcher block, then I chop strawberries on it three days later, and the chopping block still smells like the chemicals that were labeled poisonous by their own manufacturer. We are eating the poison. How safe is that?? The same is true of my dishwasher soap. And my shampoo. I didn't like any of the ingredients I was reading.

That is the journey that led me to oils. It is the story that starts after my migraines were eradicated. It is that path that showed me how seriously I needed to take clean living. You may carry this to amazing places—sourcing raw honey and grass-fed beef, growing kefir and kombucha cultures on your counter, and more—or you may simply become a dedicated oiler. There is no wrong choice. You're not better or worse than someone who has carried natural health to other places. Rest in the fact that <u>every step is a good step</u>.

Hear this: you matter. Your family matters. You may not realize how close you are to a very dangerous place with your health, or how ailments that are already going on are interconnected with the products on your cabinets or your diet. One thing I've realized is that everyone's body has a breaking point of how much it will tolerate. For some people, it metastasizes as a migraine or even daily headaches, like it did with me. For others, it's indescribable pain. For others, swelling and inflammation. For others, skin issues. For others, hormone issues. For others, depression. For others, fear and anxiety of things that never scared them before. For others, inability to sleep. For others, anger. Some of it is emotional. Some of it is physical. All of it is your body screaming for help. I am not saying that every health issue is linked to a lifestyle of toxic chemicals. But I am saying that if you've been battling something, that may not be a bad place to check. Rule it out. That simple step changed my life.

I realized quickly on my journey that food was only half the equation. There were other things that had to change in my home. Every toxic chemical I eradicated was something my family was no longer exposed to. And they were worth fighting for. Let me prepare you for one thing: in this little book, I'm not going to just hit on oils. I'm also going to touch food. It's because using an oil to masque a gut problem does not work. The two go hand in hand. You undermine a clean lifestyle if you use oils and eat poorly. Look at both, and take steps on each as you feel led.

This is where my story with oils begins. I saw the value of a toxin-free life. I learned what it truly meant to pay attention to ingredients. And this is why I can train you to do the same thing. Simply cutting toxic chemicals in our home has led to dramatic weight loss; it has eradicated eczema, sleep issues, nightmares, thyroid issues, and so many other problems. I had no idea that toxins were the root cause. They threw my system into chaos. It's not about oils fixing things. It's about dangerous chemicals damaging things. You don't have to feel the way you're feeling anymore.

It's time to make a change.

Let me talk to you for a moment about the dangers in your house, and why it's so critical that you take this seriously. This isn't intended to scare or overwhelm you, just to make you aware of what's in your cabinets. Once we've done that, I'll walk you through slow, simple steps on how to start using your kit and Young Living.

The number two cause of death in the United States is cancer. Cancer expenditures in 2011 were 88 billion dollars. 1,620 people a day die of cancer. There are 10,000 new cases a year among children. One in three cases in the U.S. is directly linked to poor diet, physical inactivity, weight, or chemical exposure. The American Cancer Society says only five to ten percent of all cancer cases are from gene defects. Five percent. That means 90-95% of cancer cases are outside our genes. It's what we allow into our homes.

The National Institute of Occupational Safety and Health studied 2,983 ingredients in our products at home and found 884 toxic ingredients. 314 of them caused biological mutations. 218 caused reproductive problems. 778 were toxic to the human body. 146 they knew caused cancer tumors—but were allowed in the United States, even though they were banned in other countries around the world. 376 caused eye and skin irritation. These chemicals are allowed in nearly every type of cleaning supplies in the United States—common things under your cabinets right now. Even organic cleaners have some known carcinogens that are just naturally derived.

26 seconds after exposure, chemicals are found in measurable amounts in the human body. The average woman applies 300 chemicals to her body a day; 80 before breakfast. The top ten most dangerous chemicals in our home are found in: air fresheners, cleaning supplies, dishwasher detergent and dish soap. Other danger spots include beauty supplies and personal care products, hairspray, gel, shampoo, and deodorant. This information is from the U.S. Environmental Protection Agency's Top 10 Killer Household Chemicals Study.

What happens when your body is chemically overloaded? You may see it in something as catastrophic as cancer. But most of us feel it in other ways; lethargy, inability to focus, sleep trouble, chronic inflammation, unexplained pain, fibromyalgia, skin issues (adult acne), hormone imbalance, hot flashes, stress, anxiety, and fear. If you face any of these issues, it's time to kick toxic chemicals to the curb.

With food, it can seem very overwhelming. You may be thinking, "Sarah, there's no way I can do that diet you did. That's INSANE." It is insane. But I was having brain bleeds every month. I needed to stop it. You may not be at that place. What I recommend for someone just starting is simple label reading. Every inch you move is an inch that will not have a hold on you anymore.

LABEL READING

This is a tip that will help you utilize Young Living's oil infused products, because it will tell you where to begin in your home. Let me start with food labels.

Perhaps you have a craving for ice cream. Ice cream in and of itself is not inherently bad, unless you're consuming it every single day. When you flip the carton over, just look at the list of ingredients. I can tell almost immediately whether it's safe for my family. Without even reading it, if the list is 30 or 40 items long, I usually put it back on the shelf. Instead of reaching for ice cream with seven different dyes, hydrogenated oils, and other yuck; go for the ice cream with milk, cream, and eggs. That's a better choice.

Look for shorter lists of ingredients with names you can pronounce. If you don't know what it is, here's a little trick I use on my cell phone in the store: type the ingredient into Google with the words "dangers of" right in front of it. (Example: "dangers of hydrogenated oils.") You'll be blown away by some of the things that you read. That's how I started this journey, by looking up ingredients one at a time.

Let me give you a quick example of label reading.

This is a popular cough drop's ingredients list: Sugar, Glucose syrup, Glucose-fructose syrup, Water, Stabilizer (Glycerol), Acids (E270, E330), Concentrated blackcurrant juice (0.26%), Flavorings, Acidity regulators (E325, E332), Emulsifier (Soy lecithin), Eucalyptus Oil, FD&C Blue 2, FD&C Red 40, Flavors.

My analysis: the first three ingredient are sugar, which we know feeds bacteria, including the bad bacteria that may be making you sick. There are at least four kinds of dye and artificial flavors that can hit your immune system. And that's just the start. You can see there's also food dyes which wreak havoc in our bodies, and several other things you may not want to ingest.

These are the ingredients in Thieves cough drops: cinnamon bark oil, clove bud oil, eucalyptus radiata leaf oil, isomalt, lemon peel oil, pectin, peppermint aeriel parts oil, rosemary leaf oil, stevia extract, water.

My analysis: oils, stevia and water! Isomalt is a sugar-alcohol that is natural and friendly to your teeth. There are no bad ingredients! This is a better choice!

The simple step of reading labels will completely change how you view everything in your house. Now let's focus on food for a moment.

I have a system I use for getting rid of all the ingredients I dislike in my food, and it's pretty simple: tackle one ingredient a week. It took me about ten weeks to eradicate most of the yuck in my diet. After that, I focused on 1-ingredient foods; like chicken, nuts, fresh fruit, or vegetables. If you can live a 1-ingredient life, you're on the right path. Our team has developed a clean living chart for eating that shows you simple steps and recommends a few books if you want to read more on this. You'll find it on the next few pages.

Week 1, Cut soy. Week 2, Cut hydrogenated oils. Week 3, Cut dyes. Week 4, Cut preservatives. Week 5, Cut nitrates from meat. Week 6, Cut all processed and pre-packed food. Week 7, Cut all sugary drinks. Week 8, Cut all corn syrup. Week 9, Cut all GMO's (genetically modified food). And Week 10, Cut gluten. I have never felt so good!

These charts are based off the teaching of Brandee Gorsline, who runs a page called Clean Living Coach on Facebook that is thousands strong. She has been my personal clean living mentor, and is a dear friend. It's also the start of the next "mini" book I'm writing on Young Living supplements. Look for it at oilabilityteam.com!

Why am I giving you information about food in an oils book? Because the two go hand in hand. You can't feel better on the outside when you are poisoning the inside. A lean living lifestyle is more than a bottle of oil or swapping out some dish soap. If you truly want to start taking steps to move past the place where you are now, you must look at diet and oils equally. I will tell you though, if this overwhelms you, skip it. Start with oils and return later. I'd rather see you implement a few tools from the book than continue where you are. My heart is to see you healthy, well, whole, and doing what you were called and created to do; without exhaustion, without pain, and in the right frame of mind. If changing your diet throws you for a loop, move to something you can take in bite size pieces—like working with your diffuser daily. You CAN do this, and it's ok to start there!

One of my frustrations with the medical system in this country is that we're always fixing things after the fact. It's about the treating of disease. What if we lived in a world where we didn't treat things, but we set the stage for our body to be strong enough to correct it on its own? What if medicine was about preventative maintenance? What if we flooded our systems with antioxidants and amino acids (NingXia Red and Aminowise), correctly sourced protein (Pure Protein Complete), greens, (Multigreens), enzymes (Essentialzyme), Omega 3's and 6's (Omegagize), probiotics (Life9) and vitamins (Master Formula), so that our body could do its work more effectively? It's not always about what you're cutting out. It's also about putting good things in. It's about building wellness one decision at a time.

Now let's go beyond your palate and break into your starter kit. I'm going to spend the rest of this book explaining why Young Living is not a hobby, but a lifestyle. You should be oiling every day, multiple times a day, in multiple ways.

Clean Living Coach

CHEAT SHEET

ORGANIC JUNK FOOD IS STILL JUNK FOOD . BEWARE OF GLUTEN-FREE FRANKEN-FOOD.

"A healthy outside starts from the inside."
-Robert Urich

"Pay the farmer or pay the hospital."

-Birke Baehr-

"Every time you eat is an opportunity to nourish your body."
-Unknown

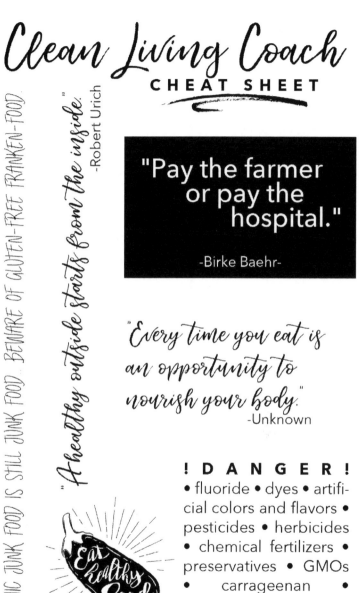

! D A N G E R !
• fluoride • dyes • artificial colors and flavors • pesticides • herbicides • chemical fertilizers • preservatives • GMOs • carrageenan •
! D A N G E R !

Clean 15

Onions
Avocado
Sweet Corn
Pineapple
Mango
Sweet Peas
Eggplant
Cauliflower
Asparagus
Kiwi
Cabbage
Watermelon
Grapefruit
Sweet Potatoes
Honeydew Melon

Dirty Dozen

Apples
Celery
Tomatoes
Cucumbers
Grapes
Nectarines
Peaches
Potatoes
Spinach
Strawberries
Blueberries
Sweet Bell Peppers
-always buy organic-

■THIS

GOOD FATS
- organic extra virgin coconut oil
- grass fed butter *(Kerry Gold)*
- avocado *(don't heat)*
- sesame *(don't heat)*
- grapeseed *(don't heat)*
- safflower *(don't heat)*
- extra virgin olive oil

GOOD SUGARS *in moderation*
- raw honey
- real maple syrup
- palm sugar
- sucanat
- stevia

SWEETENERS
- see sugars

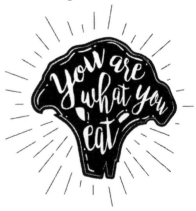

.not: **THAT**

BAD FATS
- Hydrogenated/ partially hydro. oils
- Corn oil
- Vegetable oil
- Canola oil
- Soybean oil
- Margarine
- Shortening

BAD SUGARS
- White bleached sugar
- Agave nectar
- High fructose corn syrup
- "ose," if it ends in "ose," its sugar

ARTIFICIAL SWEETENERS
- Aspartame
- Splenda
- Sweet'N Low
- Equal

GMO's
(Genetically Modified Organisms)
- Corn
- Soy
- Pineapples
- Sweet Potatoes
- Salmon
- Canola

Look for GMO-free project approved website

ENRICHED WHITE FLOUR
It's poisoning you! (pizza crust, bread, crackers, wraps, etc.)
- Synthetic B vitamins
- Reduced iron
(extrememly toxic)
- Bromine
(endocrine distruptor)

SOY
Say no to soy! (check out this book: *"The Whole Soy Story" by Dr. Kayla Daniel*)

MSG
Excitotoxin that hides under dozens of names on food labels. Causes serious neurological damage, migraines, seizures, heart palpitations, and hundreds of other symptoms
Visit msgtruth.org

MOVIES

that will change your life:

A Diet for All Reasons
A Place at the Table
A River of Waste
Beautiful Truth
Bottled Life
Cowspiricy
Death by China
Diet for a New America
Dive
Drugs Never Cure Disease
Earthlings
Eating
Farmageddon
Fast Food Nation
Fat, Sick, and Nearly Dead 1 & 2
Fed Up
Fluoride: The Hard to Swallow Truth
Food Chains
Food Fight
Food, Inc.

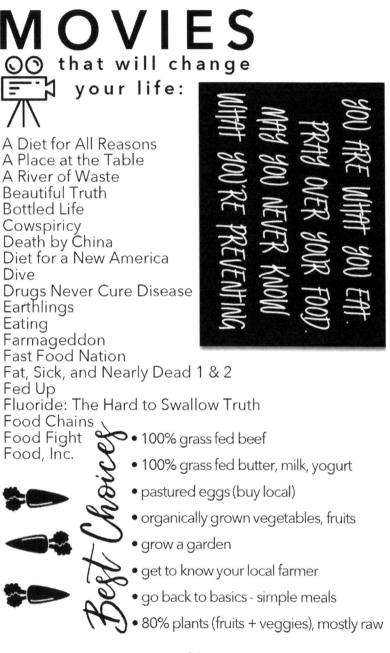

YOU ARE WHAT YOU EAT.
PRAY OVER YOUR FOOD.
MAY YOU NEVER KNOW
WHAT YOU'RE PREVENTING.

Best Choices

- 100% grass fed beef
- 100% grass fed butter, milk, yogurt
- pastured eggs (buy local)
- organically grown vegetables, fruits
- grow a garden
- get to know your local farmer
- go back to basics - simple meals
- 80% plants (fruits + veggies), mostly raw

"The food you eat can be either the safest and most powerful form of medicine or the slowest form of poison."   -Ann Wigmore

"You don't have to cook fancy or com-plicated masterpieces—just good food from fresh ingredients."   -Julia Child

"No tricks, gimmicks, special pills, special potions, special equipment. All it takes is desire and will."
-Richard Simmons

"You are what you eat, so don't be fast, cheap, easy, or fake." -Unknown

"You don't have to eat less, you just have to eat right." -Unknown

"Came from a plant, eat it; was made in a plant, don't."   -Michael Pollan

SHOPPING TIPS

- buy locally and eat seasonally
- shop the perimeter of the store
- support local farmers/markets
- buy one ingredient foods
  with no labels
    (veggies, fruits, butter, raw milk)

READ EVERY LABEL
don't eat what you can't pronounce

BOOK
RECOMMENDATION
a great place to start learning more about clean living:
Living Balanced: Healthy Mind & Body Reference Guide by Stacey A Kimbrell

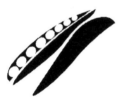

TOSS THE MICROWAVE OVEN! NUKING DESTROYS NUTRIENTS REPLACE WITH A CONVECTION TOASTER AND STOVE TOP REHEATING.

Overwhelmed?
Start simple.

Flip over the box of each thing you eat and look at the ingredients list. If you don't know what it is, Google it, with the words "dangers of" in front of the ingredient. If you want ice cream, it's not bad. Just grab ice cream with milk, vanilla, and eggs instead of icecream with 30 ingredients. The shorter the ingredients list, the better.

Where did I start?

Week 1 I cut soy.

Week 2 I cut hydrogenated oils (which cause cancer).

Week 3 I cut dyes.

Week 4 I cut preservatives.

Week 5 I cut nitrates.

Week 6 I cut all processed food.

Week 7 I cut all sugary drinks.

Week 8 I cut corn syrup.

Week 9 I cut all GMO's-- genetically modified food.

Week 10 I cut gluten. And I feel GREAT. Take it one step at a time with what you can handle.

10 weeks to a healthy diet, in baby steps. Every choice pulls you closer to feeling healthy.

-Sarah Harnisch

WHY WOULD YOU
WANT OILS IN YOUR HOME?

Oils have no yuck. They are just the steam distilled or cold-pressed oils from a plant. There are millions of uses for oils and oils infused products: to support systems in the human body like your cardiovascular system or your endocrine system for hormones, to support your joints, or your brain, or liver. They are used to replace chemical cleaning supplies. Thieves cleaner is all I use to wipe down my bathrooms, my stove, my kitchen, my floors, and it's made of plants and six essential oils. Young Living makes Thieves laundry soap, dish soap, fruit and veggie wash, wipes, and dishwasher soap.

You can use oils infused products to replace your personal care products. Young Living has an entire line of shampoos, soaps, conditioners, eye creams, face washes, and even an entire Savvy Minerals makeup line that are completely green and chemical free. If you use oil-infused supplements, you get the benefit of the supplement along with the power of the oil. Young Living has the best ingredients list for a protein powder I've ever seen. Protein is brain food. I swap protein for sugar-laden cereal each morning.

There are 100,000 chemicals on the market today. The Toxic Substance Control Act of 1976 (TSCA) grandfathered them in. What does that mean to you? Simply put: these chemicals have not had any safety testing, and we know very little information about their side effects. Of the chemicals tested, toxic labeling is only required if 50% or more of the animals tested die. Under the TSCA, manufacturers are protected by trade laws that allow them to keep their ingredients lists a secret. Dr. Samuel Epstein, chairman of the Cancer Prevention Coalition, says, "it is unthinkable that women would knowingly inflict such exposures on their infants and children and themselves if products were routinely labeled with explicit warnings of cancer risks. But they are not labeled."

Since the 1940's, prostate cancer is up 200%. Thyroid cancer, 155%. Brain cancer, 70%. Breast cancer, 60%. Childhood cancer, 35%. The American Cancer Society estimates a 50% rise in cancer rates by 2020.

There is a standard set for non-industrial buildings by OSHA for chemical exposure. The average home has an astonishing level of 50 parts per billion (ppb). That's 50 times what's allowed. The quality of air inside your home is five to seven times more toxic than outdoor air. Chemical household cleaning product sales was a 7-billion-dollar industry in 2007.

Now that I have scared the tar out of you, and you're afraid to look under your sink, let me give you some hope.

Young Living has changed my life. It's because of the mindset. They are a pioneer in the industry. When you get that starter kit, it's the beginning of a whole different way of taking care of your family.

One of the things that makes the company so unique is that it's holistic. It's not just about oils. It's about oil-infused EVERYTHING. Soap, laundry detergent, personal care products, cleaning supplies, cooking supplies, tools for working out, love for your pets, your babies, your kids... it hits every area of your life. I've never seen a company tailor its products like this one. It truly is a total lifestyle.

When you use oils, you'll see some pretty amazing things—things I can't write about in this little book, because they are not Food and Drug Administration (FDA) approved. But I can tell you Young Living has worked with some of the top labs in the world, like the National Institutes of Health, to offer FDA-approved insect repellent, pain cream, cough drops, and sunscreen. They are showing the world what oils can do. And we're getting approval from the government to say it—because it's scientifically true. As the years roll on, more and more products will be cleared for use that are oil-infused. That's something no one in the world is doing. We are the first. It's groundbreaking—just like founder D. Gary Young's work finding new oils, and just like his work designing distilleries that are copied all over the world. This company is the best of the best of the best, a pioneer in the oils world.

Maybe you have a supplement that you take every single day that you LOVE. You have taken it for decades. Here's why you should consider switching to Young Living's supplements.

All Young Living supplements are infused with essential oils. Without oils, your body's blood absorption rate is less than half of the supplement in 24 hours. With oils, it spikes to 86% in one hour. It's called bioavailability. For example, "clinical experience has shown that before putting essential oils in the Multigreens formula, there was 42% blood absorption in 24 hours. After adding the essential oils into the formula, blood absorption increased to 64% in 30 minutes and 86% in one hour. The conclusion was that the cells were now receiving nutrients that they had previously not been able to assimilate." (Essential Oils Desk Reference, 1st Edition, p. 205). That's why you want supplements infused with oils. That's why you use cleaning products with Thieves. That's why you put on deodorant infused with lemon and lavender. It's not just about wearing deodorant or cleaning without toxins.

Oils are tiny, molecularly. They carry the beneficial ingredients from supplements and other products to every cell. The oils themselves are so tiny; they act as little cars, allowing nutrients to piggy back off them to the different cells in your body. It's not about oils healing the body. It's about using them as a tool to carry good things to your body to support its systems; then letting your body do its own healing, as it was created to do.

"In 36 years of clinical practice, using a wide variety of high end nutritional supplements, I have had the best clinical results using nutritional supplements infused with therapeutic grade essential oils from Young Living. Clinical results are seen in 1/3 of the time of any other supplement I have recommended." ~Carla Green BScPT, RegAc, Young Living Diamond

It works the same with every product Young Living has: Savvy Minerals makeup, the Seedlings line for babies, the Kidscents line, diffusers, massage oils, cleaning products, supplements, the Slique Weight Loss line, the Vitality cooking line, sunscreen, insect repellant. It doesn't matter what you choose—every oil-infused product is better than what's in your cabinets right now.

You now have two very good reasons to start cleaning out your cabinets:

1) The stuff in your home is toxic, and you don't want to poison your family.

2) Even the products you have that may be relatively good are likely not oil-infused, so your body is not assimilating even half of the product. It's time to use something that does better than that.

Open that box!

Now let's shift gears so I can start giving you tools, and discuss how to play with your Young Living starter kit. This is where it really starts to get fun, and where we start to strip fear. I'm going to take you deep inside your kit, delving into the world of aromatherapy in the simplest way you've ever heard. It doesn't need to be scary. You don't need to be perfect, and you don't need to be fast. My goal is to give you passion and ideas. This is the crack-open-the-unopened-bottles-in-my-starter-kit section of the book.

Here we go.

You have the kit in your hands and you know what to do with Thieves and Pan Away, Lemon smells great in your diffuser—but what on earth is Copaiba??? And how do you say it?! (Coh-puh-ee-buh, by the way.)

My goal is to get you reaching for an oil every time you would grab a product from your home. And that takes training. You will hesitate. And that's ok. (I did too!) It took years for me to totally transform my house— so don't feel like you're not moving fast enough. Let me show you what the end result is. If you go to our website, oilabilityteam.com, and click on "share" and "free stuff," there is a video called the Oily Scavenger Hunt Video. It's what my home looked like after I started swapping all the yuck out of my cabinets. It features the Harnisch herd, my five kids. We are the real deal. I don't just tell you things without living it myself. If you need a goal to keep in front of your mind, revisit the video and stay focused. Write down your monthly oils wish list in our "Gameplanner" planning system. I show this video in my oils classes to train people on a toxic chemical-free lifestyle.

How often should you use oils? Every single day. As much as you can. The biggest mistake I see as an aromatherapist is that people aren't using oils frequently enough. I love this quote from fellow aromatherapist Jen O Sullivan: "They should be viewed as another wellness regimen upon which we embark. You don't brush your teeth or take a shower only when you feel like it. When you want results and overall wellness, you do something long-term and with deliberate dedication."

OILS SAFETY

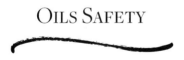

Why do we fear oils? We don't know what we're doing. We are afraid of wasting a few drops of our investment. Why do we think that? People have been using oils since Bible times without direction. God made them pretty fool-proof. I love this from Jen O Sullivan: "Today, there are hundreds of thousands of people, if not millions, using essential oils under their own supervision and without knowledge or understanding of how or what they are using. However, these people using oils on a regular basis have one thing in common: there have been no major issues with people becoming sick or dying from their use. The alarmist mentality in the aromatherapy industry on the whole is unnecessary, because people are using oils to raise their level of health and are doing it on their own. It seems as if the certified aromatherapists of the world are not too happy. And why should they be? Their would-be clients are self-diagnosing and self-treating with much success!" (French Aromatherapy).

One woman asked me on Facebook the other day if my "hokey" oils actually worked. I told her Young Living is doing 1.5 billion dollars in sales every year, and selling 50,000 to 100,000 starter kits a month. (Eddie Silcock, Direct Selling News, Starter Kits: A New Consultant's First Impression). That means they are either duping a **lot** of people, or the oils work. On our own team, we have over 40% on Essential Rewards, where they order what they choose every single month. If four in ten people on my team are re-ordering every single month, and our team does 300,000 dollars in sales a month just three years after I got my starter kit; something they order must actually work. They keep coming back.

Don't fear the oils. Just get them on or in your body. Let's talk about how to do that. Then I want you to practice, and I'll show you how get confident with your kit.

THREE WAYS TO USE THE OILS

There are three ways to use essential oils: aromatically, topically, and internally. Let's start with five aromatic uses. These are simple things that you can do in five minutes or less to break the seal on those bottles of oil.

AROMATIC USES

1) Open the cap

This is the simplest way to experience an oil. But if you open the cap and smell the bottle, it will smell differently than when it's out of the bottle on your skin or in the diffuser. Why? Because each molecule is made up of three different types of constituents—top notes, middle notes, and base notes, just like a music staff. The difference is volatility, which describes how quickly an oil rises into the air.

Top notes move the fastest. They are the first smell you get right out of the bottle, and it's the sweetest of the three smells. They almost act like a sugar rush, hitting the brain first and satisfying its desire for the smell. (It's like a mother's milk for a nursing baby—the first milk satisfies a sugar rush! God made the plants the same way.)

Base notes are out of the bottle last, like the goodness at the bottom of a mug of hot chocolate. If you want the benefits of the base notes, but don't have time to diffuse, the best way to do that is to put a drop of oil in your hand. The oil will stay intact and you'll get the top, middle, and base notes all together as one molecule.

2) Hand Cupping

This is next method is just as easy. Once the cap of the bottle is open, place a drop in your hand. Don't touch the orifice reducer (the silicone piece at the top of the bottle that allows the oil to drip out). When you touch it, you leave your epithelial cells (your dead skin cells) on the reducer. Over time it makes your oils less potent.

Place two to three drops in the palm of your non-dominant hand. Flatten your hand, then take your other hand and rotate the oils clockwise. By doing that, you're getting the molecules spinning. You know how the shape of your DNA is in a double helix, sort of like a ladder? When you spin the oils in that direction, as they enter your body, they can shoot right up your DNA. It allows the oils to enter your system faster because they are following your body's cellular makeup.

Pro-tip: rub the oils on your skin, but don't wash your hands! It's like opening your bottle and dumping the oil down the sink. It's a waste. The oil will be absorbed into your skin almost immediately without a greasy residue. My favorite place to rub my "leftovers" are on the top insides of my ears (that's an emotional point, there are lots of nerves that lead to the brain), the bottoms of my feet where my pores are large, or the back

FEARLESS

of my neck to hit my spine. Just about everything goes through the spine, so you're hitting a lot of points in the body by placing it at the nape of your neck.

3) Diffuser Jewelry

This is a beautiful and effective way to enjoy your oils! Buy a piece of jewelry that has a porous element, drip oils on it, and smell it throughout the day. Untreated wood, leather, cork, felt, and lava stones can hold an oil for four to eight hours. One of my favorite diffuser necklaces is on Lucy Libido's website, lucylibido.com.

4) Spritzers

Adding to oils to water puts them in a form that allows you to spray the oils where you want. You can a spritzer to freshen a room; to un-stink your teenager's shoes, or your dog (or dog crate); to freshen the sheets just before your guests spend the night; or as a body spray. If you are using a 2-ounce sprayer, I put about ten drops of oil in the bottom, a pinch of salt to help disperse the oils, and fill it to the top with water or witch hazel (with no alcohol). If you are using a 4-ounce sprayer, I do 15-20 drops. Honestly though, those are just loose guidelines. If your nose likes more or less, adjust accordingly.

I use amber glass bottles because oils and toxic chemicals don't mix, and plastic is a toxic chemical. The oils will go after it. (It takes a good 12 weeks for an oil to discolor a plastic bottle, but over time it will break it down). I use colored bottles because oils will break down in sunlight. If your bottle is amber-colored (or blue, or green—anything that's not clear), it will preserve the oils.

My favorite place to order supplies is Amazon if you just need a couple bottles, but if you want to teach a DIY class and need more supplies, glassbottleoutlet.com is cheap, as is Bulk Apothecary. One of my favorite books for DIY's is Jen O Sullivan's *Essential Oils Make and Takes*, and *Oil + Glass: The Must Have Essential Oil DIY Recipe Book*, by Yael Marmar and Joanna Katz. Both have hundreds of recipes if you just want to have some fun and make your own oil infused personal care products.

Now for the non-DIY'er, or the one that *wants* to be a DIY'er but legit doesn't have the time, let me give you two simple solutions. Enter the DIY kit, courtesy of Young Living. They now sell a kit where you can make an aromatic spritzer, a luxurious lotion, and a lip balm all in one neat little **DIY box** (item number 21861). All the supplies come in the kit: the bases, the containers, the labels. All you need are the oils that are in your starter kit for a crazy fun experience. There's no need to order supplies, labels, or containers. It's all in one little bundle. Play without stress.

The other option Young Living has for you is the **Thieves Cleaning bucket** (item number 20421). I LOVE this. It is one of my favorite items in all of Young Living. It comes with a little pouch filled with nearly half a dozen oils for you to try when you're cleaning, a steel cleaning bucket, a microfiber cleaning cloth, and one of the largest glass spray bottles I've ever seen with a "Thieves" label on the side. The benefit to having the bucket is that you can tinker with smells that you like during cleaning. Pine oil is included, as well as Thieves, Purification, Lemon, and Citrus Fresh. I love to use Pine and Lemon on my floors and Citrus Fresh on my kitchen and bathroom counters. I use Thieves EVERYWHERE.

5) The Diffuser

This one you can do right now, because one of these came in your starter kit! You may have the Dewdrop diffuser or the Desert Mist diffuser (with a flickering candle setting! BOOYEAH!) Or you may have been a lucky duck that ordered the Rainstone diffuser (my personal favorite) with your kit.

Why do you want a diffuser going in your home all the time? Let's break down what a diffuser does.

First, it creates a spa-like atmosphere in your home or office! The Dewdrop diffuser generates ultrasonic frequency waves at 1.7 million times per second, releasing a steady stream of essential oil molecules into the air to fill any room with an relaxing, inspiring aroma. A diffuser is one of the simplest ways to surround yourself with the aroma of essential oils because it's hands off and automatic. Plus, it's a mini humidifier. Humidified air keeps your skin moisturized and your body feeling fresh.

Second, a diffuser replaces toxins in your home. You can now eliminate odors without using synthetic air fresheners (Google the dangers of plug-ins... WOW). You can replace candles with a diffuser. Doctor Andrew Sledd, who is a pediatrician who specializes in Environmental Toxicology, said, "It takes only 1 hour of burning a candle to produce the same effects as smoking a single cigarette." Research by the U.S. Environmental Protection Agency shows candles release the dirtiest soot, sometimes containing particles of zinc, tin, and lead. Compared to a cigarette, a candle "is more dangerous because it doesn't have a filter on it, which removes hundreds of millions of micro particles," said Dr. Sledd. Sledd says the soot particles penetrate the deepest parts of the lung and could cause respiratory illness. One of the first swaps I made was to ditch the candles in every room and replace them with a diffuser and pure Young Living oils. And that was tough for me, I was a candle-holic! But toxins are toxins and I wanted them OUT!

You might think you are making a better choice by using organic candles, but many of them are just as dangerous. You may have switched to soy candles. I'd caution you strongly to get as far from soy products as possible. Soy is an anti-nutrient, it is the top hormone disruptor in the United States, and yet it is in everything—soy lecithin, hydrolyzed soy protein, etc. Hormone disruptors mean you have a hard time losing weight, among other issues. Soy is even in most chocolate! A wonderful resource on soy is Dr. Kayla Daniel's book, *The Whole Soy Story*. If you must have candles in your home, the only candles that I trust are made of 100% pure beeswax. Another great option is the Desert Mist diffuser, which has a candle setting that flickers (with the benefits of oils filling your nose!).

Finally, diffusers are another tool to safeguard your family's health. Instead of the chemicals from a plug-in air freshener or a candle, you're replacing them with a pure essential oil. You swap toxins for plants. And not just any plants. If you're using Lemon oil, for example, that oil alone has constituents that are scientifically shown to support the body's immune system. Thieves has similar properties. Every oil in the kit has benefits to different systems of the human body. This is about making small, better choices.

There are tens of thousands of diffuser recipes out there, but let me give you a few that I REALLY love to get you started:

Blends from the starter kit:
Calm and Strengthen: 3 drops Lavender + 2 drops Copaiba
Focus and Inspire: 3 drops Frankincense + 6 drops of Lemon
Relax and Wind Down: 3 drops Stress Away + 2 drops of Lavender
Wake Up with a Smile: 2 drops Lemon + 1 drop Peppermint

My favorite blends in the diffuser:
3 drops Northern Lights Black Spruce + 2 drops Geneyus
Valor
En R Gee
Oola Grow
Highest Potential
Release

Stress Away
2 drops Grounding + 3 drops Valor + 1 drop Highest Potential

My favorite single oils in the diffuser:
Cypress
Frankincense
Lemon (I could diffuse this all day long)
Idaho Blue Spruce
Bergamot (a yummy citrus!)

WHAT DO YOU PUT IN THE DIFFUSER AND HOW OFTEN DO YOU DIFFUSE?

You can run just about any combo of oils in your diffuser, but generally not more than six to eight drops of oil. Creating your own diffuser blend is simple and easy and up to personal preference. This is because each body is different, (made of a different biochemistry) and each body will want a different ratio. Your own body may want less or more, based on the day. Oils you loved yesterday may be repulsive today. Then you may crave them and return to them later. It all depends what your body was exposed to, what it's fighting, and what it wants. Your body's "oils mood" changes like a teenage girl. So always revisit old smells.

I like to mix my single oils but generally leave the blends alone, because they already have so many oils in them. Dr. David Stewart once said if you don't like an oil, carry it in your pocket for three or four days until your frequency starts to match, then smell it again and see if you like it. (By the way... Dr. Stewart's book, *Healing Oils of the Bible*, is still my favorite aromatherapy book of all time. Go grab a copy!)

How often do you diffuse? All. Day. Long. If it gets to a point where it bothers you, then your body is on overload. Just shut the diffuser off and take a 3-minute walk outside. Open a few windows. You're not getting hurt by your diffuser, your olfactory system is just on overload. Even too much water can be a bad thing. Your body will take what it wants and toss the rest. The only negative effect may be a slight headache.

What oil do you pick? Follow your nose. Your body knows what it needs. It can guide you if you take just a few moments every day to open your bottles and smell your oils! One day you may CRAVE Lemon oil. The next it may be Frankincense. And after a long day away from home, Stress Away.

I make it a point to take three minutes and try a new oil in my diffuser at least once a week. I have come up with many new favorites! The biggest tip I can give you on your diffuser is to PLAY with it. (Then make sure you write it down!) Your favorites may not be someone else's. But every time you turn it on, you're doing your body a favor.

If you can't remember to have the diffuser on all day or if you are in a work environment where you can't run one, place it in strategic spots around the house. I have one in my bathroom so I can just pop it on when I am getting ready in the morning. I have one on my nightstand for when I am reading in the evenings; or in the living room where my family gathers to watch movies together or play board games at night. I have one on my kitchen counter, ready to go with water in it, for when I get home and I'm making dinner. I place one in each of the kid's rooms with peppermint inside to tingle their noses when it's time for school. I even have an orb diffuser in my car to deal with the soccer smell from my kid's uniforms after practice, and an orb diffuser by my swing to enhance my time outdoors.

Place the diffusers where you'll use them, even if they are not on every minute of the day. Remember, the goal is to USE your starter kit. That includes your diffuser.

Challenge #1

Make it a point to try all 11 oils from your starter kit in your diffuser over the next 11 days. Then after that, start mixing and matching them to find your favorite combos. Remember to write your recipes down! After 11 days, go another 19 days repeating some of your favorite smells, or the smells you are most drawn to. It's said that anything you do for 30 days becomes a habit. Let's make it a habit of getting a diffuser going in your home every single day.

TOPICAL USES

Are you ready to get hands-on with your oils? Ready to take your oils to the next level? This section is pretty cut-and-dry. Here's my in-your-face aromatherapy instructor advice:

Get the oil on your skin.

That's as hard as this gets. Most of your learning comes through experimenting. As a certified aromatherapist, here are my thoughts on pursuing certification before beginning to use the oils: **I learned just as much by playing around with my oils and doing my own experiments as I did studying genus and species of plants during my multiple certifications**. You will learn SO much more than any certification just by getting oils on people. Every aromatherapist I have spoken with agrees. Play.

What's my advice? If you love education, educate yourself with solid aromatherapy books instead of certifications. Then tinker and play and re-create what you read. The home aromatherapist is just as legit as one with a piece of paper on their desk. I feel more knowledgeable from what I have seen laying my hands on people than anything I learned in a classroom. The science of aromatherapy is all lab work. Your home and your friends and your family are your lab. You have permission to have some serious fun.

There are a few points I want to lay down when you are talking topical application. If you master these simple tips, you will be ready to use the oils with confidence.

When and why to dilute

My rule of thumb is to always dilute with children, and always dilute the first time you use an oil on an adult. After that, I generally don't dilute unless I see redness; which can be toxins escaping the skin, a reaction with something already on your skin, you may have sensitive skin, or you may have an interaction with a pharmaceutical drug in your system (for more on drugs and oils, read Scott Johnson's, "Evidence Based Essential Oil Therapy").

The rule of thumb is to always have a carrier with you. ALWAYS. If your skin turns red, don't panic, just use a carrier oil. I always keep one handy in my purse, because I never know how my body will respond on a different day. It doesn't mean the oil is making you sick, it means it's doing what it was designed to do. You just don't want it working that fast, with your body pulling it in so quickly that your skin turns red. A carrier oil is any oil whose molecules are larger than essential oils. A few different carrier oils are olive, grapeseed, hempseed, jojoba, macadamia, and sweet almond—the favorite of aromatherapists. My personal favorite oil is V-6 from Young Living. It's a blend of six of the top carrier oils, and it's what I use on my children.

You can apply carrier oil on the skin before if you expect redness, or after—it works either way! Here's a pro tip for using carrier oils: when your starter kit arrives, the first thing to do is make a roll-on with a carrier oil in it (you can buy 10 mL roll-ons on Amazon inexpensively. I recommend the ones with the metal roller ball). I keep one in my purse, one in the car, and a few in strategic places in the house. If I ever have any type of redness, I have a carrier at-the-ready to dilute the essential oil on my skin. If you don't have access to Amazon and want to start with your kit immediately, take one of the tiny amber colored Share It bottles from your starter kit and make up a little vial of carrier oil with what you have in your kitchen. That will give you access to a carrier on day 1.

Challenge #2

Make three roll-ons with carrier oils and put them in strategic places to have them ready when you need them!

Again, how your skin responds today may not be how it responds tomorrow. And how you respond to one oil may not dictate your response to others. Keep that in mind and carry a carrier oil roll on and you can feel free to experiment!

Photosensitive Oils

There are a few oils that are photosensitive. That means you don't want to put them on your skin, then go out in the sun. Photosensitivity happens when the plant material is processed and the part of the plant that photosynthesizes is still preserved. Then, when sunlight hits it, it wants to photosynthesize on your arm! You can get a good burn by wearing those oils for prolonged periods of time in the sun.

Furanocoumarins is a compound in some oils that can greatly increase UV sensitivity. While most photosensitive oils are citrus, other oils can contain compounds or mixes of compounds that have the same effect as furanocoumarins, meaning they're not sun-safe either.

The side of the oils bottle will tell you if the oil is photosensitive and tells you to stay out of direct sunlight for 12-48 hours after applying. The oils that come in the starter kit that are photosensitive are Citrus Fresh, DiGize, Lemon, Stress Away, and Thieves.

If you accidently apply one of those oils, make sure your skin is covered if you'll be outside gardening or watching your kids play soccer. There is a wonderful color-coded chart called the "Suggested Product Claims Chart" that shows you which oils are photosensitive. You can access the chart in your virtual office on the Young Living website, under "member resources" and "product education."

While I'm on the topic of your Virtual Office—do you know what that is? Young Living has an entire website of your whole history with the company. You can look at your orders, place Quick Orders, get on the Essential Rewards program to start earning free oils, see if anyone has signed up under you, check out your paycheck, and learn a LOT about the company with the wonderful "Getting Started" videos.

Challenge #3

If you're brand new to Young Living, snag your username and password, go to youngliving.com and click "sign in"—and click the "getting started" tab right on the front page. There are several short videos that illustrate Seed to Seal (where your oils came from!), Young Living, your personal team, and more. It's where I began when my kit showed up on my doorstep. If you don't know your username and password, you can call Young Living Member Services and they will help you out. Watch all the short Getting Started videos to complete this challenge!

Uncomfortable Spots

There's one more thing to tell you about topical application: Be careful where you place oils. If you're just starting out, stick with the feet to start—they have the largest pores on the body, and yet the skin is tough. I have a little word mnemonic that I share with my team: go low and go slow. Start on your feet (low) and dilute if you're unsure or uneasy. Once you're comfortable with an oil, use it other places.

Don't ever place oils inside the ears, in private areas, or near eyes. It can be very, very uncomfortable. If that ever happens, use your V-6 oil and dilute immediately by rubbing it all over the skin that was exposed. Don't flush your eyes with water; what do you know about oil and water? They don't mix. Use a carrier oil instead.

Favorite Ways of Using Oils Topically

Some of my favorite places on the body to place essential oils are on my big toes (that's where the nerve endings come out for your brain), on my chest, under my third and fourth fingers (that's where the nerve endings come out for your sinuses), over my heart, anywhere on my feet or hands, on my spine, on the inside of the top of my ear (but never in the ear hole where the eardrum is), and on the back of my neck.

You can be strategic about where you place the oils, or you can slather them just about anywhere and get benefits. If you're unsure of where to place them, start with your hands and feet. That's where most of your nerve endings come out, and you'll hit a lot of points by beginning there. If you want to be more purposeful, look up "Vitaflex Points" on Google for images of those nerve endings in your hands, feet, and spine, and place the oils in those spots. Remember our rule of thumb: "go low and slow." Start with the feet and use less oil then you think you will need. You can always add more oil later.

Challenge #4

To get you confidently using your starter kit, apply an oil to-night in a place where you've never applied one. It might be on the mastoid bone behind your ear or your big toe. You might talk your spouse into a massage to get some Stress Away on your spine or the bottoms of your feet. Next week, try a new spot.

I started giving hand massages to my kids each night before bed with Lavender oil. I'd go about five minutes and gently rub the oil into their skin. I found after a few nights with five kids, at least one would get back in line and try to trick me into giving a second hand massage! It was a great way to bond with my kids. There are many 5-minute tutorials on hand and foot massages on YouTube. Even if you learn one small technique, like gently pulling the ends of the fingers, it can be very relaxing.

Don't know which oil to apply topically? Use the same trick I showed you with the oils in your diffuser: smell a few of them and see which one your body wants. You'll be surprised—it won't always be the same oil.

More topical techniques

Now let's dig into some deeper aromatherapy. If you are getting pretty comfortable trying new places on the body for your oils, let's pull our attention off "where" you are placing them and more onto "how" you do it.

This where you can really start to get the most out of your kit.

There are two types of topical application in the aromatherapy world: layering and blending.

Layering is when you put each oil on your skin right out of the bottle. You may lay down Stress Away, then Lavender, then Citrus Fresh, one right after the other. If you wait 30 seconds before applying the next oil, it gives your body a chance to use it more effectively. This requires no preparation, just some down time with your starter kit. You can come up with some pretty fantastic recipes just by playing around.

How do I make up layering combos?

It just comes with an awareness of your needs. Maybe you're falling asleep one night and notice that you broke a nail. Look up a nail bed support recipe the next day and try laying the oils on your fingers. Every time you're thinking of something that's bothering you, make note and see what's out there in the essential oils world that may support that system. Chances are, it's already been thought of.

I keep a checklist of things I see on my kids or my husband or my family, and then do a little digging to see if there is something in the essential oils world for what I see. I am amazed at the millions of uses of oils every single time I delve in. There are hacks for things as simple as DIY Citronella Floating Candles to Lavender lemonade (on the Young Living blog)!

Here are some of my favorite resources for new recipes to try:
   The Young Living blog (which has won awards!) at www.youngliving.com/blog/
   French Aromatherapy, by Jen O Sullivan
   Conquering Toxic Emotions, by Rhonda Favano (we'll talk more about this later)
   The Art of Blending with Essential Oils, by Debra Raybern

Gentle Babies: Essential Oils for Pregnancy, Child Birth and Infant Care, by Debra Raybern

Essentials: 50 Answers to Common Questions About Essential Oils, by Dr. Lindsey Elmore

The Essential Oils Desk Reference, 7th Edition, by Life Science Publishing

There's An Oil For That: A Girlfriend's Guide To Using Essential Oils Between The Sheets, by Lucy Libido (don't worry—it's rated G!)

The Chemical Free Home 1, 2, and 3, by Melissa Poepping

Healing Oils of the Bible, by Dr. David Stewart

My two favorite sites to pick up Young Living-friendly aromatherapy books:

Life Science Publishing (discoverlsp.com)

Growing Healthy Homes (growinghealthyhomes.com)

Blending is a fun technique that saves time when you want to use multiple oils together. You can use blends for perfumes, skin care, massages, your favorite diffuser oils premixed, salves, and ointments. I also make Vitality blends ahead of time in a single bottle to make it easier to put together recipes I use frequently.

There are only three real rules to blending: put it all in the same bottle, write down what you did, and let it sit for at least 24 hours. That allows the oils to meld together.

Let me give you an example.

When I need some support for my respiratory system, I love to use Thieves Vitality, Oregano Vitality, and Frankincense Vitality. It looks something like this: 10 drops of Thieves Vitality, 8 drops of Oregano Vitality, and 2 drops of Frankincense Vitality in a veggie capsule. If I plan on using that recipe for a while, it saves me time to make a blend.

I will put the following into a bottle and let it sit for a day:

100 drops Thieves Vitality

80 drops Oregano Vitality

20 drops Frankincense Vitality

Then when I go to place it in a veggie capsule (find these on Young Living's website), it's already premixed and I can just fill the capsule up without trying to grab multiple bottles and open the caps while I have a veggie cap filled with oils in my other hand. It's the simple way to get multiple oils on or in your body.

Another good use for blending is night-time oils. Each of my kids has a certain set of oils they love to use every single night. I make up their mix and blend it, and it's easy for me to apply to their chest and feet each night. I mix the blend up with V-6 so it already has a carrier in it, ready for their skin.

Challenge #5

Make up your own blend, and place it in a strategic place in the house so you will remember to use it! Find a need your family has—maybe it's a relaxation blend for bedtime. Maybe it's a blend to soothe your feet after a long walk. Pro tip: Once you have your first empty bottle, you can recycle it as a container for a custom blend! No waste! Let's piggy back off this challenge of getting oils on your body and kick it up a notch.

I also want you to think of 3 things you'd like to tackle with your body over the next month. Maybe you could use Cool Azul Pain cream for relief from minor muscle and joint aches, arthritis, strains, bruises, and sprains. Perhaps you'd like to try Young Living's Thieves cough drops to relieve coughs, sooth sore throats, and cool nasal passages. Make it a point to list 3 things you want to tackle this month, and add those products to your order. Next month, make a new list and start over.

Back to topical training: I also like to make some of my own skincare products. I love eye serums that you dot around the outside of your eyes. I'll pick a carrier oil like grapeseed oil, which is good for facial skin, and add Frankincense, Lavender and Myrrh to it. (Don't do Peppermint near your eye! It's unpleasant!)

I also have a blend for mental clarity that I use almost daily, especially when I am writing books. That blend has 8 drops of Northern Lights Black Spruce, 4 drops of Geneyus, and 2 drops of Brain Power. It's one of my favorite blends to diffuse! (Just multiply that recipe by ten if you want to fill a 10mL bottle).

How many drops fit in a bottle? A 15mL bottle will hold 250-300 drops. A 5mL bottle will hold 85-100 drops. The empty 2mL amber glass drams that came in your starter kit will hold 34-40 drops (about one third to half of one of your 5mL bottles of oil), and the sample sachets hold four to six drops.

While we're on the topic of bottles, I have another challenge for you!

Challenge #6

The empty-the-box challenge. There are so many of us that open the box, smell all the oils, and get distracted and ignore everything else inside! I want you to get the most out of your investment, so here's how to do that and complete this challenge:

Use your Share It amber colored bottles, and share oils with people in your life. Give them just a few drops of the oil in one of the sample bottles. I want you to completely wipe your stash of bottles out. You have been given such a special gift in a toxin-free lifestyle with Young Living! Share it with those around you! (If three of them buy a Premium Starter Kit using your distributor number, which you can find in the Virtual Office under "my organization," you are paid $50 per person! Three people would equal a check that would cover the cost of the starter kit you purchased!)

Drink those two red packets! They are NingXia Red. And they are the best thing in the box! My favorite way to drink them is cold—so pop them in the fridge first, then try them out in the afternoon when you could use a nutritional boost! NingXia Red is made of berries grown in the NingXia region of China. (If you don't know how to read that word, don't sweat it. I studied Japanese and it threw me for a loop too! It's pronounced "Ning-shah", though some call it Ninja juice!) It's loaded with antioxidants that you want in your life!

Read every piece of paper. Legit. Sit down with all those papers in the front of the box. Young Living has an amazing story. If you want to learn even more, the whole history of this amazing company, all the way down to the seeds that founder D. Gary Young hid in his boots to start his first farm? It's on your virtual office under "Quick Order," and it's called "D. Gary Young, World Leader in Essential Oils." Knowing the story behind this amazing company will empower you to use them with confidence!

You have a big playground ahead of you, friend. There is so much to try! This whole section has been about erasing fear and replacing it with passion and ideas. I think we've accomplished that! But just in case you're still intimidated by all your kit has to offer, let me tell you how to do this each day without feeling overwhelmed. Pick a different thing to try at least once a week. Make up a blend. Try a few new oils in your diffuser. Make up a face serum. Layer a new oil. Most of what I learned came from simply getting the oils on my body and the bodies of my friends and family around me. That's how you can become fearless with the oils: begin using them each day with the tips in this book.

I also make it a point each month, even as a Young Living Diamond, to try one new oil I've never used. As of this publication, there are 82 single oils bottled by Young Living. There are 81 blends, six massage oils, four roll-ons, and 12 different oils collections. By my math, if you tried just one new oil a month, it would take you 15.4 years to try them all!

Challenge #7

Order at least one new oil each month on your Essential Rewards order! Never be afraid of new things—delve in! Your starter kit came with a knockout cool catalog of every single oil Young Living has. One of the first things I did when it showed up was to go through that catalog and circle every single product I thought my family would use. Then I organized them by priority, got on Essential Rewards to earn points as I tried new items, and I was off and running.

Here's a pro tip: my first goal when I got my starter kit was to double my oils collection as fast as I could. We'd had the kit for a week and had already seen it work on our family over 80 times. I wanted to get as many oils as possible in my home! But I only had 20 dollars a week to live on after our mortgage, gas, utilities, food, and debt. So I got the cheapest thing I could find: the Golden Touch Kit. That kit has seven oils in it for 89 dollars wholesale—that's just a little over $12 a bottle. The only other oils that cheap on from Young Living are their Vitality oils. In a month, I'd nearly doubled my collection just with that one kit! And I had seven new oils to try, without breaking my budget.

Another great way to get new products in your home is to consider sharing the oils. You'll fall madly in love with them as you start swapping things in your home. If you'd like to learn more about how to get your oils for free, grab one of my other mini books, *Your Gameplan*, off Amazon or our website at oilabilityteam.com. Purchasing the Premium Starter Kit was the best financial decision of my life. It has completely changed my life. If you truly love the ideas in this little book and you ache to get more oils in your home, snag my other mini book. It will give you direction and focus on how to get your oils for free. I have never paid for a single oil I own—they were all free through essential rewards or from my paycheck. I even used my first check to pay my husband back for my Premium Starter Kit. We have never looked back.

INTERNAL USES

We have gotten to the hum-zinger. This is the one that scares the tar out of new oilers. It's the topic of most controversy. If you Google it, you'll see many, many posts against internal use. Let's start by wiping away fear.

All of the oils in Young Living's Vitality line have GRAS (Generally Regarded As Safe) status from the Food and Drug Administration, which means Vitality oils are approved as food additives. You can put them in food and drinks and safely consume them at reasonable doses. Every GRAS oil has a well-documented history of safe use. For a food substance to meet GRAS specifications, the following four criteria must be met:

-the substance has to be recognized as safe by experts
-the experts have to be well trained
-safety must be scientifically proven
-the FDA must know the intended use of the food

When GRAS experts go to evaluate a food additive, like Grapefruit Vitality oil in your water, they work through a rigorous test set. For an essential oil to reach GRAS status, they look at: 1) toxicology—at what strength does the essential oil become poisonous to a child? 2) Organic chemistry—what is the chemical makeup of the oil? 3) Biochemistry—how will the chemistry of the oil interact with the chemistry of a human? 4) Metabolism—what path does the oil take through the body and how is it absorbed? 5) Pathology—what illness or disease would be caused if a human was poisoned?

Many of the Vitality oils in Young Living's collection are names you know: Basil, Cinnamon Bark, Clove, Copaiba (the elusive South American oil returns!) They have been used for centuries in food.

Since the oils have been through toxicology, chemistry, biochemistry, and metabolic testing—and have a long history of being safe, I am comfortable using Vitality oils in my home. Tens of thousands of Young Living members order and safely use Vitality oils every single month.

How to Take Oils Internally

Keep in mind, the only oils designated for safe use internally are the ones in the white Vitality bottles. I cannot safely recommend other Young Living oils for internal use. I cannot recommend ANY non-Young Living oils for internal use because no other company offers the Seed to Seal guarantee of purity and potency that Young Living does.

My favorite way of using the oils is as a "bomb" or "bullet". That's a few drops of Vitality oil in a clear veggie capsule. The capsules are sold on Young Living's website, and dissolve as vegetable when they hit the gut. Size 00 capsules will hold about 16 drops. If your stomach reacts to the oil, try making an entire capsule of carrier oil first, like V-6. It will dilute the oil when it hits your stomach and make it easier to break down.

Here is a Vitality recipe that I love to use:

Adrenal Support: equal parts of Basil Vitality, Peppermint Vitality, and Nutmeg Vitality (3-4 drops each in a capsule)

(flip back to the section on blending for my respiratory support recipe!)

Other ways to use Vitality oils:

-add 2 scoops of Vanilla Pure Protein complete to water or milk with 5 drops of Orange Vitality for a Dreamsicle-flavored morning shak!

-mix frozen ice (1 cup), berries (1 cup), raw honey (4 tablespoons), vanilla yogurt (1/2 cup), Pure Protein Complete (2 scoops) and NingXia Red (2 ounces) in a smoothie with 2 drops of Tangerine Vitality

-make NingXia Red shots. I love this recipe from Young Living: 1 ounce of NingXia Red, 2 drops of Tangerine Vitality and 2 drops of Lime Vitality

-baste your meats in Basil, Lemon, or Black Pepper Vitality oils (after cooking them)

-drop a few drops of Oregano, Basil, and Marjoram Vitality oils into your spaghetti sauce right before you serve it

-add a drop of Thieves Vitality to your hot chocolate or morning coffee

-try replacing herbs and spices in your favorite recipes with Vitality Oils. Some of the Vitality herbs are: basil, cinnamon bark, fennel, ginger, oregano, rosemary, and thyme. There are also Vitality mint oils like peppermint and spearmint, and vitality citrus oils like lemon.

Challenge #8

Make one of the Vitality recipes above! You get double points if you replace your morning coffee or sugary cereal or frozen breakfast sandwich (or if you are skipping breakfast) with a Pure Protein Complete smoothie!

I am not a gourmet chef, but I love to play with the oils in my kitchen. It really takes your homemade treats up a notch! We've done some neat things to pancake and brownie batters, and baked goods; and added citruses to many a dish and many a drink to infuse it with flavor.

Keep in mind that the oils are volatile, meaning they want to leap into the air. If you add heat, volatility happens even faster. Try adding the oils at the end, just before you serve the dish. When putting your oils in water, use a dispersant like Himalayan salt. (You only need a pinch—not enough to change the taste of the water.) Again, remember what you know about oil and water? They don't mix. The oil molecules will cling to the salt granules and help them disperse throughout your drink.

One of my favorite books on cooking with Young Living oils is *A Chef's Guide for Cooking with Essential Oils*, by my dear friend, Jason Pilkington. He has an entire conversion chart in his book so you know exactly how much oil to use when you're trying out your own recipes. Young Living also has an incredible cookbook called, *From Our Fields to Your Table*, (Item number 5689). I have tried every recipe in the book. Both books are incredible and take "playing with your oils" to a whole different level!

EMOTIONAL OILS

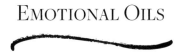

This is one of the most commonly under-used aspects of oiling, simply because most people don't understand how much the oils can impact our brain and emotions. With permission, here is a quote from the book, *Conquering Toxic Emotions*, by fellow Diamond and dear friend Rhonda Favano:

"Unresolved emotional experiences are recorded in cellular memory, DNA, and remain there as live programming until they are dealt with. These unresolved emotions can be stored anywhere within the human body.... The definition of emotions are any feelings of joy, sorrow, fear, hate or love, etc... and any strong agitation of the feelings... are usually accompanied by certain physiological changes, such as increased heartbeat or respiration, crying or shaking."

This is key to understand: emotions can cause physiological changes! I experienced this myself when I was almost in a car accident about two years ago. My vehicle and the driver's car in front of me never touched, but the fear of what could have happened in a near head-on collision at 60 miles an hour with all five of my kids in the car stuck with me. After ten minutes, my heart was still racing, my palms sweaty, and I was lightheaded and delirious. There was a direct connection with the stress and memory of something that never even happened—and a physical response from my body. Even now when I think of that incident, my heart rate speeds up. Years later, my body remembers it.

Rhonda goes on:

"You may experience stress, tension, anxiety, depression, chaos, and other negative feelings without considering how they affect you emotionally and physically. These negative feelings lower your body's frequency and the body's electrical system. This weakens the body's ability to fight off infection, sickness, and disease. Negative thinking can lead your mind into toxic thinking, which has a serious effect on your body."

The best advice I can give you on emotional uses of oils is simply to get the oils on your skin or in your diffuser again and again and again and see how you feel. Often when I am frustrated, I pop an oil in my diffuser only to realize hours later that the rest of my evening went smoothly. Play and see how you feel.

Not only does Young Living have cleaning supplies, supplements, and kid's products, they also have emotional oils. If you have a hard time letting things go, if you can't seem to shake grief, or bad memories haunt you, or struggle with certain emotions and reoccurring cycles of negativity, it may be worth looking into the Feelings Kit. The names of the oils are self-explanatory: Harmony, Release, Inner Child, Forgiveness, Present Time, and Valor. The Ancient Romans used some of the oils found in the Valor blend for bravery before heading into battle. I love Harmony in my diffuser when I start my school day. I put Forgiveness on my children's feet just after I break up a fight and we need to have a heart to heart. I use Present Time to keep my eyes focused on what's ahead, instead of dwelling on old problems. My favorite uses of the kit are to put the oils on my feet, hands, and spine topically; and to diffuse them during the day. The smaller the room, the more concentrated the oils will fill the room.

HOW TO KEEP LEARNING

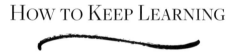

We have hit on a LOT in this little book. You now know about all the major oils topics in one small space. And you have a list of challenges to teach you to start reaching for oils first. Every time your hand goes to a cabinet for something you once used, pause and ask yourself if there is an oil you can use instead.

The most important step in going toxin-free is being willing to keep learning and to look things up! Google is your friend! Whenever I have a question, I type it into the Google search bar with the words "Young Living". For example: "Young Living relaxation." I get great ideas! I also like Life Science Publishing's, *Essential Oils Desk Reference*, and the search bar on the website pubmed.com (a medical research site) when I have oils questions. Before you contact the person that helped you get your kit, always try those places first! Learning to research will be one of your greatest tools in oiling.

Challenge #9

Make a list of three things you'd like to work on for support of your family's health this month. Look up oils to support certain systems of the body—either on Google, with a reference guide, or on pubmed.com. Practice the simple art of research! It's amazing how many things you can answer on your own, just with the click of a mouse, for free!

What are the other rules we went over? If you get a headache, take a short break and get some fresh air. If you have redness on the skin, use a carrier. If you do not notice a change from what you are doing, you may not have used enough oil. People often ask me for the exact amounts of oils to use, but it really depends on your body chemistry and what you have been exposed to. One day, one drop of lemon in your diffuser may smell strong to you, and the next, five drops is hardly enough. You have to go by what your body wants. It sounds strange, but your body will talk to you. Smell the oils and see what it's drawn to.

What on earth do you do with all this information?? This is about 50 years of aromatherapy all tucked into one tiny little book! Just remember: Start slow. Start small. Start with what you are most convicted on. The goal first is to use the oils you already have. So accept my challenges and break open the bottles. You may fall madly in love with an oil you've never smelled. Or you may hate it—until you put it in the diffuser and fall in love with it there!

Here's a quick list of just some of the uses for the oils Premium Starter Kit. Eleven oils. Thousands of uses. This list is not by any means comprehensive, but it will give you a few ideas.

Copaiba:
Rub on your chest to elevate your mood
Apply to your temples to slow down a racing mind
Inhale in cupped hands for mental clarity
Rub on legs that are overworked
Apply a small amount to your lips when there is cold wind
Diffuse for focus and calming emotions

Frankincense:

Drop on the back of the neck as a natural perfume
Diffuse at bedtime for calm and relaxation
Smell a drop in cupped hands to promote positivity
Take Vitality Frankincense internally for immune support
Use on face to moisturize and support your skin (Frankincense is used
  in the Young Living ART skin care line)

Lavender:

Inhale in cupped hands for relaxation
Add to Epsom salt for a relaxing bath
Try Lavender Vitality oil for respiratory support
Hair health--add it to your Young Living shampoo
Apply on the stomach when nervous
Add to shea butter for a soothing skin balm
  (or add it to the Young Living DIY kit!)
Add to the dryer on a small cloth to make your linens smell amazing!

(Check out the Lavender Calming Bath Bombs (item 20671) WOWSA!)

Lemon:

My favorite for surface cleaner—
  I put extra lemon oil in the Thieves cleaner
Use Lemon Vitality to rinse produce
Use to get sticky goo off things
Apply to the feet before wearing high heels
Diffuse for uplifting atmosphere
Works as a stain-stick for clothing

Peppermint:

Has a cooling effect on the body,
  apply to the back of the neck when it's hot
Can assist in mental alertness
Stimulating when smelled straight from the bottle
Diffuse for kids who are trying to do homework
Settling when rubbed on the abdomen

DiGize:

Rub on your stomach after a big meal
Use DiGize Vitality oil in a capsule to support healthy digestion
Inhale to feel re-energized

PanAway:

Use before and after physical activity

Energizing and cooling to muscles

Add to a carrier oil for a soothing massage

Apply to the tailbone to warm up before any activity

Rub on tired feet at the end of the day (my favorite use!)

Rub on the neck, shoulders, and temples to release tension

Apply to the knees for a warming sensation

Purification:

Add to baking soda for a carpet freshener

Put one drop in smelly shoes

Great to add to Thieves laundry soap or dryer balls

Combine with coconut oil to support your skin

Diffuse daily to get rid of pet smells, a house of boys, sports, or dirty laundry

Add to a cotton ball and place in air vents

R.C.:

Mix with V6 for a soothing chest rub

Use it for a relaxing massage

Inhale in cupped hands to ground your emotions

Rub on your chest and back before an early morning workout

Place a few drops in the bath or shower

Apply to your chest and wrists for uplifting

Stress Away:

Relaxing and calming as a perfume

Diffuse for a peaceful sleeping environment

Use as a linen spray

Roll on before shopping with kids

Apply to the temples

Helps with "butterflies"

One of my favorite oils to diffuse in the car (the ORB diffuser is great for the car, item 5227!)

Great for crowds of people or uncomfortable situations

Thieves:

Great cleaning power and an irresistibly spicy scent

Refresh musty carpets

Diffuse for feelings of peace and security

Helps to eliminate odors

Thieves Vitality supports a healthy immune system

Add a drop of Thieves Vitality to oatmeal, granola, cereal, or hot drinks

Add Thieves Vitality to a veggie capsule as a daily supplement

That wraps up our tour of the Premium Starter Kit, and this mini book on becoming fearless with Young Living essential oils!

Something in this book hit you in the gut. Something convicted you. I want you to begin in that place. Perhaps it was the way that you eat. Cut one ingredient a week. Perhaps it was the laundry soap in your cabinets right now or the cleaning supplies under your sink. (Did you know that Thieves cleaner costs $1.50 per spray bottle to use? One container of Thieves cleaner is concentrated and makes over 20 spray bottles to replace glass cleaner, floor cleaner, bathroom cleaner and a spray for your counters. It's very affordable! It's the first item I tell my team to put on their essential rewards order right after they get their Premium Starter Kit). Maybe you are convicted about the shampoo in your shower. Perhaps it is your morning routine, which is completely empty of real nutrients to start your day—and you want to incorporate Pure Protein Complete.

Here's the thing: there's no wrong way to start. You're not wrong if you try just one new thing. You're not wrong if it takes years to get some of the things out of your home. It's not a race.

But every decision you make is better than staying where you are.

If I could slip into your home and train you how to use your kit today, I'd say just <u>open the bottles</u>. Even if you are not sure how to use them, open them and be brave. Apply an oil before bed. Apply three different oils during your day tomorrow. Carry them with you, and see how you feel. Keep a couple of Vitality oils at the dinner table, and pass them throughout the whole meal. See if you can go through an entire dinner without the oils sitting on the table for longer than two minutes. Put an oil you have never diffused in your diffuser. Creatively make your own blends.

You get better at using oils when you strategically place them all around the house in the spots you would utilize them. That brings me to

Challenge #10

The 3-cabinet challenge, the last challenge in the book. I have given this challenge in over 800 classes nationwide, and now, it's your turn.

After you close this book, pick three cabinets in your home, and grab your favorite products. These are the items you've cleaned with for years, the soap you have used since you were a teenager, your favorite sauces in your pantry, or the favorite smell you burn or plug in day after day after day. Flip those items over. Look at the labels. If you don't know what a word is, look it up on Google with the words "dangers of" in front of the ingredient. Some of the products in your home right now will blow your mind!

Then start small. Do what I call the "simple swap." It doesn't need to be an entire room at a time, or even multiple products. Pick what bothers you the most, sign up for essential rewards and commit to kicking toxic chemicals out of your home, one month at a time. At the end of the book, I'll make the simple swap even simpler for you by breaking it down room by room with checklists so you can pinpoint some of the danger zones in your house.

WHAT IS ESSENTIAL REWARDS?

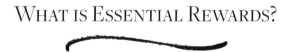

I keep mentioning Essential Rewards, but I haven't fully explained it. Essential Rewards is like Christmas every month. These are Young Living products—oils, supplements, cleaning supplies, personal care products, makeup, Slique weight loss products, kid's products, diffusers, massage oils, deodorant and more; that you select and order every month You can change the date it ships each month. You're not locked in to the same order. You can cancel it anytime with no fee. Oh—and because you already have your Premium Starter Kit, you get wholesale pricing at 24% off… for life.

What are the benefits to Essential Rewards?

Free oils. From the first moment you order, you get 10% off your order as rewards points. That means if you spend 100 personal volume (PV), you get a 10-dollar bottle of oil for FREE. That's a free bottle of Lime or Cedarwood for ordering Laundry Soap and Thieves Cleaner and swapping dangerous chemicals from your cabinets. If you log into your Virtual Office at youngliving.com, you can see how many points you have at any given moment that can be used for free product whenever you choose.

After three months, you get 20% back on your essential rewards orders. After 25 consecutive months, Young Living gives you 25% back! You're getting paid to order your laundry soap, dishwasher detergent, and shampoo. No grocery store I know does that on every single purchase. And I've never seen a store give 25% back on every single order—no strings attached. No yearly fees. No membership costs. This is the most cost-effective way to kick the toxins out of your home with the simple swap. Young Living is a generous company that is committed to coming alongside us and making the Simple Swap affordable.

On top of the rewards, *you can also earn free oils every month*. By spending either 190PV , 250PV, or 300 PV (most items are dollar for dollar for PV), you can earn free oils. For example, the Essential Rewards bonus oils for the month of August 2017 were five of the six Kidscents collection oils: Geneyus, SleepyIze, TummyGize, Owie, and SniffleEase; as well as Clarity, Citrus Fresh, Envision, and Lemon. The value was $266.46 on a $300 order. If you want those oils twice, most months you can place a second 300PV order on Quick Order and get another $266 in free oils, to use August as an example. You can get the promos twice, once on Essential Rewards and once on Quick Order.

Essential rewards is worth it. It's how I grew most of my oils collection. If you are serious about toxin free living, this is exactly where I would start. The minimum order to keep your Essential Rewards account active is 50PV a month, or $12.50 a week. You can cover that out of your regular budget simply by swapping cleaning supplies, shampoo, and toothpaste that you already buy at the store. But your new Young Living toothpaste has no yuck!

Log into your virtual office using your username and password, the one you set up when you got your kit (call Young Living Member Services at 1-800-371-3515 if you do not remember your password). Click on the "Essential Rewards" button, and start the simple swap. Pick out the products you want you switch over first. If you need a place to write it down, use the white space in this book.

Swapping out toxins is not a joke. It's your life. It's the lives of your family. It's my passion to show you how to do this, after suffering from migraines for 24 years because of the dangers in my home. I will never go back! I know where that road leads. It's time to make a change. Toxic chemicals have no place in your house.

Try all ten challenges to build confidence with your kit. Here they are again so you can check them off in one easy place. When you complete each challenge, put the date next to it. When you have all ten done, go to oilabilityteam.com/fearless/ and I'll have a free download just for you!

□ *Challenge #1*

Make it a point to try all 11 oils from your starter kit in your diffuser over the next 11 days. Just one oil a day, you can do it! When you are done, make up your own blends and try those. See if you can run your diffuser every day, even if it's just a few minutes, for 30 straight days to build a habit of diffuser use.

□ *Challenge #2*

Make three roll-ons with carrier oils and put them in strategic places! Now you're ready to use oils topically on yourself, kids, or your friends!

□ *Challenge #3*

Watch all the short videos under the Getting Started tab in your virtual office at youngliving.com. If you want me to give you a tour instead, go to oilabilityteam.com, click on "Start Here," "Gameplan Bootcamp" and "Day 6: Your Greatest Tool: A Detailed Tour of the Young Living Virtual Office." My tour is free!

□ *Challenge #4*

Apply an oil tonight in a place where you've never applied one. (I recommend getting your spouse or a friend to giving you a Stress Away back massage!)

□ *Challenge #5*

Make up your own blend. Put it in a small Share It bottle from your kit or recycle your first empty bottle from your kit! If you want to kick it up a notch, focus on 3 areas of your wellness regimen, make a list, look up products that may support those areas, and give them a try. Each month focus on 3 new things.

☐ Challenge #6

Empty-the-box challenge! Use all your Share It bottles to share oils with friends and family. Drink those two red NingXia packets. (Be brave! It's berries!) Read all the literature and smell all the oils!

☐ Challenge #7

Order at least one new oil each month! See how quickly you can double your oils collection! Start swapping yuck out of your cabinets for oil-infused products!

☐ Challenge #8

Make a Vitality recipe! You get bonus points if you try a Pure Protein Complete smoothie in place of your regular breakfast using a Vitality oil!

☐ Challenge #9

Practice the art of research. A good oiler knows how to look things up. Make a list of three things you'd like to work on to support your family's body systems this month and piggyback off challenge 5. You CAN do this.

☐ Challenge #10

The Simple Swap or 3-cabinet challenge. Pick 3 items in your house that you're the most convicted to swap out, get on Essential Rewards, and start taking small steps to clear out every toxic chemical from your home.

You can do this, one room at a time. Take up the challenges. Start the Simple Swap. Connect with the person that gave you this book. Get plugged into their classes and attend Young Living rallies near you to learn about new products, get farm updates, meet founders Gary and Mary Young, and connect with other oilers. We're all on an oily adventure together.

Young Living was one of the best decisions of my life! I no longer have fear or guilt over what's in my home. Instead, I have relief and satisfaction that I am protecting my family from the dangerous ingredients that I used to use. You will never look back. Use the graphics in this book to guide you. If you want a large print version, you can download the simple swap pages for free at oilabilityteam.com/fearless/.

Young Living is on the cutting edge when it comes to infusing your life with oils. If you loved this book and feel empowered, continue learning by checking out my website at oilabilityteam.com. There are dozens of FREE interviews at Young Living Farms and with corporate, more ideas for Essential Rewards, my books, free audio lectures, and DVD's and CD's that I have written and recorded to train you on oils. I'm also on Facebook every Tuesday night at 8PM Eastern to answer your questions in a roundtable format at Oil Ability with Sarah. Tens of thousands of oilers join me there every Tuesday.

Apply Stress Away. Take a deep breath, and dive in. You have GOT this. You are not alone. You CAN make the simple swap. Your pace is perfect. Your choices and convictions, correct. You can't mess this up—because every choice is a good choice.

Just begin.

You now have the knowledge to be fearless with essential oils!

the Simple Swap

26 SECONDS
AFTER EXPOSURE, CHEMICALS ARE FOUND IN MEASURABLE AMOUNTS IN THE HUMAN BODY.

The National Institute of Occupational Safety and Health studied 2,983 ingredients in our products at home

- **884** toxic ingredients
- **314** caused biological mutations.
- **218** caused reproductive problems.
- **778** were toxic to the human body.
- **146** cause cancer tumors

Take it one room at a time!

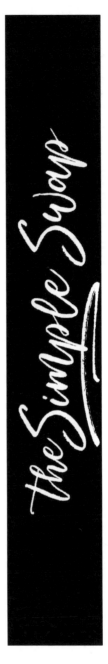

the Simple Swap

Laundry

- laundry detergent
- fabric softener
- stain spray
- stain stick
- bleach

Kitchen

- dishwasher detergent
- counter spray
- dish soap
- hand soap

Cleaning Closet

- dusting spray
- carpet cleaner
- toilet cleaner
- mirror/window spray
- floor cleaner
- air freshener
- cleaning wipes

Supplements

- immunity
- daily vitamins
- brain and heart
- allergies
- probiotics
- hormones
- fish oil
- digestive issues

Beauty Care

○

- facewash
- toner
- moisturizer
- lotion
- eye cream
- makeup
- makeup remover
- deodorant
- brightener cream

Bathrooms

○

- shampoo
- conditioner
- facewash
- bodywash
- toothpaste
- dental floss
- mouthwash

Baby + Kids

○

- diaper rash cream
- baby oil
- baby wipes
- lotions
- vitamins
- kids shampoo
- kids body wash
- kids toothpaste
- enzymes

Etc.

○

- suncscreen
- bug repellant spray
- cough drops
- pain cream
- energy boosters

TAKING IT ONE ROOM AT A TIME

the Simple Swap

LAUNDRY

Laundry detergent •	Thieves Laundry Soap	5349
Fabric softener •	(wool dryer balls + essential oils)	
Stain spray •	Thieves Household CLeaner	3743
Stain stick •	Thieves Household Cleaner	3743
Bleach •	Thieves Household Cleaner	3743

KITCHEN

Dish soap •	Thieves Dish Soap	5350
Hand soap •	Thieves Foaming Hand Soap	3674
Dishwasher detergent •	Thieves Dishwasher Powder	5762
Counter spray •	Thieves Household Cleaner	3743

CLEANING CLOSET

Dusting •	Thieves Household Cleaner	3743
Carpet cleaner •	Thieves Household Cleaner	3743
Mirror/window spray •	TThieves Household Cleaner	3743
Toilet cleaner •	Thieves Household Cleaner	3743
Floor cleaner •	Thieves Household Cleaner	3743
Air freshener •	Desert Mist Diffuser	21558
Cleaning wipes •	Thieves Wipes	3756

SUPPLEMENTS

Immune system •	NingXia Red	3042
Daily vitamins •	Master Formula	5292
Allergies •	Allerzyme	3288
Brain/heart health •	MindWise	4747
Probiotics •	Life 9	18299
Hormone sypport •	Progessence Plus Serum	4640
Fish oil •	Omegagize	3097
Digestive support •	Essentialzyme	3272

BEAUTY CARE

Facewash •	ART Gentle Cleanser	5361
Toner •	ART Refreshing Toner	5360
Moisturizer •	ART Light Moisturizer	5362
Eye cream •	Wolfberry Eye Cream	5145
Brighterner cream •	Sheerlume´	4833
Makeup •	Savvy Minerals	varies
Deodorant •	AromaGuard Deodorant	3752
Lotion •	Hand & Body Lotion	5201
Makeup remover •	YL Seedlings Baby Wipes	20428

BATHROOMS

Shampoo •	Copaiba Vanilla Shampoo	5194121
Conditioner •	Copaiba Vanilla Conditioner	5195121
Facewash •	ART Gentle Cleanser	5361
Bodywash •	Bath & Shower Gel-Sensation	3748
Toothpaste •	Thieves AromaBright Toothpaste	3039
Dental floss •	Thieves Dental Floss	4464122
Mouthwash •	Thieves Fresh Essence Mouthwash	3683
Kids bathroom •	see Baby + Kids	

BABY + KIDS

Baby lotion •	YL Seedlings Calm Scent	20438
Baby oil •	YL Seedlings Calm Scent	20373
Baby wipes •	YL Seedlings Calm Scent	20428
Diaper rash cream •	YL Seedlings Diaper Rash Cream	20398
Kids shampoo •	KidScents Shampoo	3686
Kids bodywash •	KidScents Bath Gel	3684
Kids toothpaste •	KidScents Slique Toothpaste	4574
Kids lotion •	KidScents Lotion	3682
First Aid Kit •	KidScents Oils	varies
	(TummyGize, Owie, GeneYus, Sleepylze, SniffleEase)	
Diffusers for kids:	Dolphin Reef Ultrasonic Diffuser	5333
	Dino Land Ultrasonic Diffuser	5332

ETC.

Sunscreen •	Mineral Sunscreen Lotion	20667
Deet bug repellant •	Insect Repellant	20701
Cough drops •	Thieves Infused Cough Drops	5670
Pain cream •	Cool Azul Pain Cream Relief	5759
Energy boosters •	Ningxia NITRO	3064

GET YOUR PRINTABLE VERSION OF

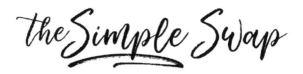
the Simple Swap

oilabilityteam.com/simpleswap

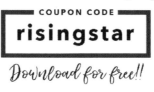

Exclusive coupon code for being a <u>Gameplan</u> fan!

COUPON CODE
risingstar

Download for free!!

designed by **OILS+CO.**

Want to learn more about essential oils and all Young Living has to offer?

Visit OilAbilityTeam.com
Home of the Gameplan System

Everything you need to confidently share essential oils, get your oils for free, and make a serious income with Young Living!

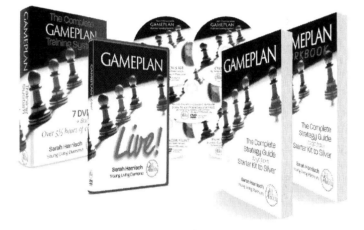

- Video and audio classes
- Printable tools & resources
- Free Business Bootcamp

- Books, CDs and DVDs
- Gameplan gear
- Shareable graphics

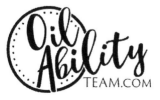

Made in the USA
Columbia, SC
27 September 2017